Fast Mimicking Diet Cookbook for Women Over 40

A Beginner's 5-Step Plan to Support Hormonal Balance and Energy, with Sample Recipes and a Meal Plan

copyright © 2025 Mary Golanna

All rights reserved No part of this book may be reproduced, or stored in a retrieval system, or transmitted in any form or by any means, electronic, mechanical, photocopying, recording, or otherwise, without express written permission of the publisher.

Disclaimer

By reading this disclaimer, you are accepting the terms of the disclaimer in full. If you disagree with this disclaimer, please do not read the guide.

All of the content within this guide is provided for informational and educational purposes only, and should not be accepted as independent medical or other professional advice. The author is not a doctor, physician, nurse, mental health provider, or registered nutritionist/dietician. Therefore, using and reading this guide does not establish any form of a physician-patient relationship.

Always consult with a physician or another qualified health provider with any issues or questions you might have regarding any sort of medical condition. Do not ever disregard any qualified professional medical advice or delay seeking that advice because of anything you have read in this guide. The information in this guide is not intended to be any sort of medical advice and should not be used in lieu of any medical advice by a licensed and qualified medical professional.

The information in this guide has been compiled from a variety of known sources. However, the author cannot attest to or guarantee the accuracy of each source and thus should not be held liable for any errors or omissions.

You acknowledge that the publisher of this guide will not be held liable for any loss or damage of any kind incurred as a result of this guide or the reliance on any information provided within this guide. You acknowledge and agree that you assume all risk and responsibility for any action you undertake in response to the information in this guide.

Using this guide does not guarantee any particular result (e.g., weight loss or a cure). By reading this guide, you acknowledge that there are no guarantees to any specific outcome or results you can expect.

All product names, diet plans, or names used in this guide are for identification purposes only and are the property of their respective owners. The use of these names does not imply endorsement. All other trademarks cited herein are the property of their respective owners.

Where applicable, this guide is not intended to be a substitute for the original work of this diet plan and is, at most, a supplement to the original work for this diet plan and never a direct substitute. This guide is a personal expression of the facts of that diet plan.

Where applicable, persons shown in the cover images are stock photography models and the publisher has obtained the rights to use the images through license agreements with third-party stock image companies.

Table of Contents

Introduction	**8**
What Is the Fast Mimicking Diet?	**10**
Why It Matters for Women Over 40	11
Safety Considerations and Who Should Avoid It	13
Understanding Hormonal Shifts After 40	**15**
Common Hormonal Changes	15
How Diet Impacts Hormonal Health	16
Signs Your Body May Benefit from FMD	18
The Basics of the Fast Mimicking Diet (FMD)	**21**
How the FMD Works	21
The Science Behind It	23
Benefits for Metabolism, Energy, and Inflammation	25
The 5-Step Beginner's Plan	**28**
Step 1: Prep Your Mindset and Pantry	28
Step 2: Understand Macro Targets and Calories	33
Step 3: Choose the Right Foods and Supplements	38
Step 4: Plan Your 5-Day Cycle	42
Step 5: Refeeding and Transitioning Back	45
Supporting Hormonal Balance Through Lifestyle	**50**
Sleep, Stress, and Recovery Tips	50
Light Movement and Exercise Guidelines	53
Tracking Energy, Mood, and Progress	55
Sample Recipes and Meal Plan	**58**
Key Ingredients to Stock	58
5-Day Sample FMD Meal Plan	60
Refeeding Day Recipes	62
Quinoa and Veggie Bowl	62
Lentil and Sweet Potato Soup	63
Avocado Toast with Eggs	64

Chickpea and Spinach Salad	65
Grilled Salmon with Steamed Asparagus	66
Greek Yogurt with Berries and Nuts	67
Veggie and Egg Scramble	68
Sweet Potato and Black Bean Bowl	69
Cauliflower and Kale Stir-Fry	70
Roasted Vegetables with Quinoa	71
Spinach, Mushroom and Feta Omelette	72
Baked Cod with Lemon and Garlic	73
Roasted Chickpea and Veggie Wrap	74
Cucumber and Avocado Salad	75
Grilled Chicken with Mashed Cauliflower	76
Turkey and Veggie Lettuce Wraps	77
Zucchini Noodles with Pesto	78
Shrimp and Guacamole Stuffed Bell Peppers	79
Lentil and Kale Stew	80
Baked Eggplant Slices	81
Avocado and Chickpea Toast	82
Stuffed Portobello Mushrooms	83
Lentil, Cucumber, and Dill Salad	84
Grilled Zucchini with Goat Cheese	85
Roasted Carrot Soup	86
Turkey and Avocado Salad	87
Sweet Potato Breakfast Bowl	88
Sautéed Green Beans and Almonds	89
Mediterranean Tuna Salad	90
Roasted Beet and Arugula Salad	91
Grain-Free Veggie Tacos	92
Quinoa and Herb Salad	93
Vegetable Lentil Stir-Fry	94
Baked Sweet Potato Wedges	95

Eggplant Caponata	96
Chickpea and Herb Couscous	97
Grilled Shrimp Salad	98
Cucumber and Tomato Salad	99
Vegetable Soup	100
Healthy Berry Parfait	101
Tips for Customizing to Your Needs	102
Final Tips and Encouragement	**104**
Staying Motivated After the First Round	104
Listening to Your Body	106
Building a Long-Term Wellness Approach	107
Conclusion	**110**
FAQs	**113**
References and Helpful Links	**116**

Introduction

For women over 40, maintaining good health can sometimes feel challenging. Hormonal changes, a slower metabolism, and the increased risk of chronic conditions often make it harder to feel balanced and energized. However, there's an effective way to support your body, improve hormonal health, and encourage longevity without needing to completely forgo food. The Fast Mimicking Diet (FMD) is a thoughtfully crafted eating plan that delivers small, nutrient-dense meals while replicating the health benefits of traditional fasting.

Developed by Dr. Valter Longo, one of the leading longevity researchers, the FMD goes beyond traditional fasting by triggering powerful processes like autophagy (cellular cleanup) and ketosis (fat-burning). By adhering to a five-day low-calorie, plant-based meal plan, women can experience benefits tailored to their unique health needs after 40. The FMD can help balance hormones, reduce inflammation, improve energy, and support sustainable weight management. It's also proven to rejuvenate cells and enhance mental clarity, offering a fresh start for both body and mind.

In this guide, we will talk about the following:

- What Is the Fast Mimicking Diet?
- Understanding Hormonal Shifts After 40
- The Basics of the Fast Mimicking Diet (FMD)
- The 5-Step Beginner's Plan
- Supporting Hormonal Balance Through Lifestyle
- Sample Recipes and Meal Plan
- Final Tips and Encouragement

Keep reading to learn more about how the Fast Mimicking Diet can help you achieve your health goals and support your overall well-being. By the end of this guide, you will have all the information and tools necessary to successfully incorporate the Fast Mimicking Diet into your life and see positive results.

What Is the Fast Mimicking Diet?

The Fast Mimicking Diet (FMD) is a scientifically designed eating protocol that mimics the effects of fasting while still allowing you to eat small amounts of food. It was developed by Dr. Valter Longo, a leading researcher in longevity and cell regeneration. The diet typically spans five days and involves eating low-calorie, plant-based meals that are low in protein and sugar but high in healthy fats and essential nutrients.

Unlike traditional fasting, which requires you to abstain completely from food, the FMD allows certain foods to be consumed in accurate proportions. These meals trick the body into thinking it is fasting, initiating similar benefits like cellular rejuvenation, reduced inflammation, and fat loss.

During FMD, the body enters a state of ketosis, which means it starts burning fat for fuel. This triggers autophagy, a natural process where the body cleans out damaged cells and regenerates new, healthier ones. The structured five-day program alternates between restricted calorie intake (usually around 1,100–800 calories daily) and nutrient-dense mini-meals, ensuring sufficient energy to function while reaping the effects of fasting.

Why It Matters for Women Over 40

Women over 40 face unique health challenges due to hormonal shifts, slower metabolisms, and increased risk of chronic illnesses. The Fast Mimicking Diet offers specific advantages for this demographic by addressing these issues head-on.

1. **Supports Hormonal Balance:**

    After 40, changes in estrogen and progesterone can lead to symptoms like weight gain, fatigue, and mood swings. Research suggests fasting-like strategies can improve insulin sensitivity and regulate blood sugar levels, contributing to better hormonal balance.

2. **Helps with Weight Management:**

    The metabolic rate naturally slows as we age, making it easier to gain weight. The FMD encourages the body to burn fat for energy, which aids in safe and sustainable weight loss without sacrificing muscle.

3. **Boosts Cellular Health and Longevity:**

    By promoting autophagy and reducing oxidative stress, the FMD supports anti-aging at a cellular level. This process helps remove dysfunctional cells and allows for regeneration, promoting better skin, energy levels, and overall vitality.

4. **Improves Gut Health:**

   A diet rich in plant-based, fibrous foods (a primary feature of the FMD) nurtures beneficial gut bacteria. A healthy gut is key to better digestion, a stronger immune system, and reduced inflammation.

5. **Encourages Mental Clarity:**

   Many women over 40 experience brain fog due to hormonal shifts. The FMD enhances ketone production in the brain, which is a more efficient energy source, improving focus and cognitive function.

6. **Reduces Risk of Chronic Diseases:**

   The diet's effects on inflammation and insulin resistance can lower the risk of conditions like diabetes, heart disease, and even certain cancers. These benefits make it an excellent choice for preventative health.

The Fast Mimicking Diet offers a range of benefits tailored to the unique health needs of women over 40, from hormonal balance to improved longevity and mental clarity. Addressing key challenges of aging, it promotes overall vitality and reduces the risk of chronic diseases.

Safety Considerations and Who Should Avoid It

While the Fast Mimicking Diet is beneficial for many, it's not suitable for everyone. Here are some key safety considerations:

- *Calorie Restriction Risks*: The diet involves a substantial cut in daily calories. If done incorrectly or for extended periods, it can lead to fatigue, dizziness, or nutrient deficiencies. Always follow the guidelines closely and consult a healthcare provider to ensure you're meeting your unique nutritional needs.
- *Pregnancy and Breastfeeding*: Women who are pregnant or breastfeeding require higher caloric and protein intake to support the child's development and milk production. Therefore, the FMD is not recommended during these stages.
- *Medical Conditions*: Individuals with diabetes, heart conditions, or a history of eating disorders should approach the diet with caution, as it may interfere with their health management plans. Similarly, those undergoing cancer treatment or with compromised immune systems should avoid fasting-like routines unless guided directly by a physician.
- *Underweight Individuals*: Those who are significantly underweight or have a history of malnutrition should

skip restrictive eating plans to avoid exacerbating health problems.

- ***Extended Fasting Risks***: The FMD should not be followed for more than five days at a time, and it should not replace regular nutritious eating in the long term. Over-fasting can harm metabolism, disrupt hormones, and deplete muscle mass.

By understanding and addressing these precautions, women over 40 can explore the benefits of the Fast Mimicking Diet safely and effectively. Always listen to your body and work with a healthcare professional to decide if this diet aligns with your lifestyle and health goals.

Understanding Hormonal Shifts After 40

Navigating the hormonal changes that come with your 40s can feel overwhelming, but understanding these shifts and how to support your body through diet can make a world of difference.

Common Hormonal Changes

Reaching your 40s can often feel like stepping into uncharted territory when it comes to hormones. The natural aging process brings about significant hormonal changes that can impact everything from your mood to your metabolism. Here are some key hormonal shifts women experience during this life phase:

1. ***Decline in Estrogen and Progesterone***: As women near menopause, declining estrogen and progesterone levels can cause symptoms like irregular periods, hot flashes, mood swings, and reduced bone strength. These hormones are crucial for menstrual regulation, bone health, mood stability, and heart protection.

2. ***Fluctuations in Cortisol***: Cortisol, often referred to as the "stress hormone," can also become imbalanced. Chronic stress or a disrupted sleep cycle during this phase of life may lead to elevated cortisol levels, which can contribute to weight gain (especially around the belly), fatigue, and difficulty managing stress.
3. ***Changes in Insulin Sensitivity***: Decreasing estrogen levels can also affect how your body processes glucose. Lower estrogen often leads to reduced insulin sensitivity, making it easier for blood sugar levels to spike. This shift increases the chances of weight gain and even the risk of more serious conditions like Type 2 diabetes over time.
4. ***Lowered Testosterone Levels***: Drops in testosterone, while less discussed in women, can also occur. This can result in decreased libido, lowered energy levels, and a decline in muscle mass, making weight management more challenging as you age.

These hormonal shifts are normal, but their symptoms and effects can be mitigated with the right lifestyle adjustments, particularly when it comes to your diet.

How Diet Impacts Hormonal Health

What you eat plays a vital role in how well your body navigates these hormonal changes. Although hormones are influenced by many factors, diet emerges as one of the most powerful tools to regulate them and manage symptoms. Here's a closer look at how this works:

1. ***Nutrient-Dense Foods***: A diet rich in whole, unprocessed foods provides the vitamins and minerals your body needs to support healthy hormone production. For example, foods high in magnesium, zinc, and vitamins B6 and D can help balance estrogen and progesterone levels. Leafy greens, seeds, and fatty fish are some excellent options.
2. ***Healthy Fats are Key***: Hormones rely on healthy fats for synthesis. Avocados, nuts, seeds, olive oil, and omega-3-rich foods like salmon can provide the building blocks for hormones while helping regulate inflammation.
3. ***Balanced Macronutrients***: Striking the right balance of protein, fat, and carbohydrates is essential for stabilizing your blood sugar and, in turn, managing insulin levels. Lean proteins and complex carbs (like quinoa and sweet potatoes) help curb sugar spikes that throw hormones off balance.
4. ***Reducing Sugar and Processed Foods***: Excess sugar and highly processed foods can lead to increased cortisol levels and worsen insulin resistance, fueling hormonal chaos. Cutting back on these and opting for whole foods can significantly improve energy levels and reduce unwanted weight gain.

5. ***Supporting Gut Health***: A healthy gut is integral to hormone health. Foods high in fiber and probiotics, such as vegetables, fruits, fermented foods, and whole grains, improve digestion and support the gut microbiome, which plays a crucial role in metabolizing and balancing hormones.

By tailoring your diet to include these elements, you can lay the foundation for better hormonal health and mitigate the more challenging symptoms associated with aging.

Signs Your Body May Benefit from FMD

The Fast Mimicking Diet is particularly helpful for addressing some of the key symptoms that arise from hormonal shifts after 40. Here are some signs that your body might benefit from incorporating this eating protocol into your lifestyle:

1. **Weight Gain, Especially Around the Midsection:**

    If you've noticed that it's become harder to maintain your weight despite following healthy eating and exercising habits, this could be linked to hormonal imbalances. The FMD promotes fat burning through mild ketosis and helps regulate metabolism, making it easier to shed stubborn weight.

2. **Persistent Fatigue:**

    Struggling with low energy levels and feeling tired, no matter how much you sleep, could signal that your body needs a reset. The FMD activates cellular rejuvenation and boosts energy production, leaving you feeling revitalized.

3. **Brain Fog:**

    Difficulty focusing, forgetfulness, or feeling mentally "stuck" could be related to decreased estrogen levels. The FMD encourages the production of ketones, which serve as a cleaner energy source for the brain, improving mental clarity.

4. **Difficulty Managing Blood Sugar Levels:**

    If you frequently experience sugar crashes, cravings, or elevated blood glucose, it may indicate a need for better insulin regulation. The FMD helps improve insulin sensitivity by lowering sugar and carb intake and teaching your body to use energy more efficiently.

5. **Chronic Stress and Poor Sleep:**

    High cortisol levels from prolonged stress or trouble sleeping can wreak havoc on your hormones. The FMD's anti-inflammatory properties and its ability to reset the body's stress response make it an excellent option for those looking to regain balance.

6. **Inflammation or Joint Pain:**

    Hormonal changes can increase inflammation in the body, leading to everything from joint pain to a higher risk of chronic disease. By supporting cellular health and initiating autophagy, the FMD helps reduce inflammation and mitigates these risks.

When combined with a healthy, balanced lifestyle, the Fast Mimicking Diet ensures that your body gets the periodic reset it needs to manage the challenges that come with aging. If you're noticing any of these signs, it may be time to consider how this structured eating protocol can complement your health goals.

The Basics of the Fast Mimicking Diet (FMD)

By now, you're probably wondering exactly how the Fast Mimicking Diet works and why it's considered so effective. This chapter breaks down the structure, science, and key benefits of FMD in simple terms, helping you understand how it can transform your health.

How the FMD Works

The Fast Mimicking Diet is a carefully structured eating plan that mimics the state of fasting while still allowing you to eat. Unlike traditional fasting, where no food is consumed, the FMD allows small amounts of specific nutrients to trick your body into thinking you're fasting. Here's how it works:

1. **Calorie Restriction:**

   The diet typically lasts for five consecutive days, during which calories are significantly reduced to around 1,100 calories on Day 1 and approximately 800 calories on Days 2–5. Calorie intake is low enough to induce fasting-like changes in the body, but not so low that you feel overly deprived or unable to carry out daily activities.

2. Macronutrient Composition:

The FMD focuses on a specific ratio of macronutrients. Meals are designed to be low in protein and carbohydrates while being high in healthy fats. This macronutrient balance triggers the body's metabolism to shift away from glucose (sugar) for energy and start utilizing fat stores and ketones, a hallmark of fasting.

3. Plant-Based Whole Foods:

The foods recommended in the FMD are primarily plant-based and nutrient-dense. Common ingredients include nuts, seeds, olives, soups, and teas. These not only provide essential nutrients but also help suppress hunger.

4. Five-Day Structure:

The five-day duration is key to achieving the diet's benefits. Shorter periods may not allow enough time for your body to enter the desired fasting-like state. A typical schedule could look like this:

- ***Day 1***: Approximately 1,100 calories to signal the body to begin transitioning to fat-burning mode.

- ***Days 2–5***: An average of 750–800 calories/day to sustain the fasting-like state and activate deep cellular changes.

By the end of the five days, your body has gone through profound metabolic and cellular improvements, leaving you more energized and better equipped to manage the effects of aging.

The Science Behind It

The Fast Mimicking Diet leverages your body's natural processes to repair, cleanse, and rejuvenate. While the science can seem complex, this section breaks it down to show how FMD supports cellular cleanup, fat burning, and anti-aging—simple and fascinating.

1. **Autophagy (Cellular Cleanup):**

   Autophagy is a natural process where cells clean themselves by breaking down and recycling damaged components. During the FMD, calorie restriction and nutrient shifts push your body into an enhanced state of autophagy. This allows your cells to regenerate and function more efficiently, clearing out harmful debris that can accelerate aging.

2. **Ketosis (Fat-Burning Mode):**

   When your body doesn't have immediate access to glucose (its primary energy source), it switches to burning stored fat, producing ketones as an alternative fuel. The FMD helps your body enter this mild state of ketosis, which is not only effective for fat loss but also provides clean energy for the brain, enhancing mental clarity.

3. **Reduced Insulin and Glucose Levels:**

   Consuming fewer calories and carbohydrates during the FMD helps reduce insulin production and lowers blood glucose levels. Over time, this can improve insulin sensitivity, making it easier to maintain healthy blood sugar.

4. **Decreased IGF-1 Levels (Aging Marker):**

   Insulin-like Growth Factor 1 (IGF-1) is a hormone associated with aging. Elevated levels promote cell growth, but they can also accelerate the aging process and increase cancer risk. Studies show that FMD lowers IGF-1 levels, which is key for slowing cellular aging and extending longevity.

5. **Anti-Inflammatory Effect:**

   Chronic inflammation is linked to conditions like diabetes, arthritis, and cardiovascular issues. The FMD helps reduce levels of inflammatory markers in the body, lowering your overall risk of disease.

6. **Stem Cell Activation:**

    During the fasting period, the body activates stem cells to repair damaged tissue and create healthier, stronger cells. This regeneration process is particularly beneficial after Day 5 of the FMD, as your body enters a rejuvenation phase.

By harnessing these natural biological processes, the FMD provides a safe and proven way to reset your body and support long-term health.

Benefits for Metabolism, Energy, and Inflammation

Women over 40 experience unique challenges when it comes to metabolism, energy, and inflammation. Luckily, the Fast Mimicking Diet addresses these concerns in several impactful ways:

1. *Improved Metabolism*: Many women over 40 notice their metabolism slowing down, making it harder to maintain a healthy weight. The FMD stimulates fat-burning while preserving lean muscle, resetting metabolic processes, and helping the body utilize energy more efficiently. By improving insulin sensitivity, it also curbs sugar cravings and reduces the risk of weight gain from blood sugar spikes.
2. *Boost in Energy Levels*: During the FMD, your body transitions from relying on glucose to burning stored

fat and ketones, which are a cleaner and more stable source of energy. This shift not only enhances physical energy but also sharpens mental clarity, leaving you feeling alert and focused by the end of the five days.

3. **Reduced Chronic Inflammation**: Hormonal changes after 40 often lead to higher levels of inflammation, which is linked to joint pain, fatigue, and a higher risk of chronic diseases. The nutrient-dense, anti-inflammatory foods encouraged on the FMD, combined with its cellular rejuvenation processes, help combat inflammation and foster a healthier, more balanced internal environment.
4. **Support for Hormonal Balance**: Because the FMD reduces insulin and cortisol levels, it aids in regulating the hormonal fluctuations that often accompany midlife. This can alleviate symptoms like mood swings, bloating, and sleep disturbances, making it especially beneficial for women navigating perimenopause or menopause.
5. *A Sustainable, Long-Term Approach*: Unlike restrictive diets that require drastic changes to your daily lifestyle, the FMD is completed periodically (typically once a month). This supports your body's natural cycles without the need for continuous dieting, making it easier to sustain.

The Fast Mimicking Diet offers a science-backed framework for addressing some of the most pressing health challenges women face after 40. With a deeper understanding of its mechanics and benefits, you're prepared to integrate this powerful tool into your wellness routine.

The 5-Step Beginner's Plan

Starting the Fast Mimicking Diet can feel like a big step, but with the right approach, you'll be fully prepared to maximize its benefits. This five-step plan will guide you through everything you need to know, from setting yourself up for success to making a smooth reentry into regular eating.

Step 1: Prep Your Mindset and Pantry

Before you start, you need to set yourself up for success both mentally and physically. Approaching the Fast Mimicking Diet (FMD) with preparation and intention can make the difference between a smooth experience and one that feels daunting. Proper planning not only ensures a more enjoyable five days but also helps maximize the benefits of the diet. Here's how you can set the foundation for success:

Set Your Intentions

Take a moment to reflect on why you're choosing the FMD. Is it to regain energy? Reset your metabolism? Manage weight more effectively? Connect the diet to a larger purpose in your life. Understanding the "why" behind your choice will serve as a powerful motivator when challenges arise.

- *Write it down*: Grab a journal or even a sticky note and jot your goals. For example, "I'm doing this to feel more energized and confident in my body" or "I want to reduce inflammation and improve my overall health." Place this reminder somewhere visible, like your fridge, pantry, or mirror, to stay focused.
- *Envision the outcome*: Visualize how you'll feel after completing five days. Picture yourself with clearer thinking, a lighter body, and a strong sense of accomplishment. This mental preparation creates a mindset of success from the start.

Consider turning your intention-setting into a ritual. Perhaps light a candle, do a short meditation, or spend a few minutes affirming your commitment to the process. This makes the start of your FMD feel purposeful and empowering rather than restrictive.

Prep Your Pantry

A well-stocked pantry is essential for staying on track. Removing temptation and organizing your kitchen ensures you aren't scrambling for alternatives mid-fast. Follow these tips to prepare effectively:

1. *Declutter and filter*: Clear out snacks, sugary treats, or processed foods that don't align with the plan. If others

in your household aren't participating, designate a separate space for tempting items to avoid accidental indulgence.
2. *Make space*: Dedicate a specific area in your fridge or pantry for FMD ingredients. Keep everything organized and easily accessible to reduce mealtime stress.
3. *Focus on FMD-friendly staples*: Stock nutrient-dense, low-calorie foods such as:
    - <u>Vegetables</u>: Zucchini, spinach, kale, cauliflower, mushrooms, and broccoli.
    - <u>Healthy fats</u>: Avocados, nuts (like almonds or macadamia nuts), seeds (chia, flax), and olive oil.
    - <u>Soups and broths</u>: Low-sodium vegetable or miso broth for comforting, warming meals.
    - <u>Teas</u>: Herbal teas like chamomile, mint, or green tea to curb hunger and aid hydration.
4. *Plan your portions*: Pre-pack portions into containers or bags, so you know exactly how much you'll eat each day. This keeps you from accidentally exceeding calorie limits.

Invest time grocery shopping a day or two before starting your FMD. Making lists with items grouped by food category can help you stay organized while shopping.

Gather the Right Tools

To simplify the process, having the right tools on hand will keep meal prep efficient and stress-free.

- *Measuring tools*: Invest in a kitchen scale to ensure portion sizes are accurate. Use measuring cups or spoons to divide out ingredients in line with the diet guidelines.
- *Meal prep containers*: Opt for stackable, compartmentalized containers to store meals and snacks for different days. This prevents last-minute confusion and keeps you consistent.
- *Blender or food processor*: These are especially helpful for preparing smoothies, soups, and other easy-to-digest meals.
- *Reusable water bottles or thermoses*: Adequate hydration is key during the FMD, so having reusable bottles around encourages frequent water or tea consumption.

If cooking isn't your forte, prep meals in bulk before you start. For instance, dice vegetables ahead of time, make broths in larger quantities, or prepare simple dishes like zucchini noodles that can last several days in the fridge.

Inform Your Support System

Having encouragement and understanding from others makes a huge difference. Whether it's your spouse, your kids, a friend, or even an online wellness group, sharing your plan helps keep you accountable and supported.

- *Be specific about needs*: Explain to family or housemates that you'll be focusing on specific meals and sticking to your plan for five days. Politely request they refrain from offering tempting treats.
- *Find a buddy*: Consider teaming up with a friend who is also looking to explore the FMD. Having someone to share tips, challenges, and wins with can make the experience more rewarding.
- *Join an online group*: There are plenty of forums and social media communities where you can connect with women who've tried the FMD. Hearing success stories and sharing your progress builds momentum and confidence.
- *Prepare for social situations*: If your FMD overlaps with events where food is a focus, plan in advance. Bring an FMD-friendly snack, such as a handful of nuts or herbal tea, so you can still participate without veering off course.

This preparation phase is an opportunity to show yourself care and dedication. By setting a strong foundation, you'll begin the FMD feeling focused, organized, and ready. Think of this as an empowering investment in yourself. For five short days, you'll be giving your body the reset it deserves and taking a meaningful step toward better health. Take a deep breath, remind yourself of your "why," and feel confident knowing you're fully prepared to begin this exciting new chapter!

Step 2: Understand Macro Targets and Calories

The Fast Mimicking Diet (FMD) isn't just about reducing calories; it's about creating the perfect macronutrient balance to drive your body into a fasting-like state while still nourishing it. Hitting these targets ensures you experience the full range of benefits, from fat-burning and cellular rejuvenation to improved energy levels and reduced inflammation.

Why Macronutrient Balance Matters

During the FMD, your body is tricked into believing it's fasting, even though you're consuming small, nutrient-rich meals. This happens because of the precise balance of macronutrients in your diet:

- *Healthy Fats (40-50% of calories)*: Fats provide a steady, long-lasting source of energy without spiking insulin levels. They ensure your body enters ketosis, where fat becomes the primary fuel source instead of glucose.
- *Carbohydrates (30-40% of calories)*: Low, controlled carb intake prevents blood sugar spikes and supports

hormonal balance. When carbs are minimized, your body transitions from relying on glucose for energy to burning stored fat instead.

- **Protein (10-15% of calories)**: Protein is kept intentionally low because high protein can stimulate growth pathways and increase levels of IGF-1 (a hormone associated with aging). By lowering protein, the FMD helps trigger autophagy, the cell-cleaning process that supports longevity.

This balance shifts your metabolism, increases fat-burning efficiency, encourages cellular cleanup, and protects against aging-related diseases. Striking the right macronutrient ratio is not just critical to the success of the FMD; it's what sets it apart from other calorie-reducing diets.

Calorie Targets for Each Day

To make the most of the FMD, follow a structured calorie and macronutrient plan over the five days:

1. **Day 1 (Higher Calories):**

    Start with approximately 1,100 calories. This allows your body to begin transitioning into a fasting-like state without feeling too deprived.

    - ***Example macros***: Fat (40-50%), Carbs (30-40%), Protein (10-15%).

- **Purpose**: This calorie level helps ease your system into the metabolic shift and prevents a sudden drop in energy.

2. **Days 2-5 (Lower Calories)**:

   Consume around 750-800 calories per day while maintaining the same macronutrient ratios.

   - **Purpose**: These lower-calorie days deepen the fasting-like effects, activating fat-burning, cellular repair, and autophagy.

Tips for Tracking and Hitting the Right Ratios

Precision is key on the FMD. Here's how you can successfully manage your calorie and macronutrient targets without feeling overwhelmed.

- *Use a Food Scale and Kitchen Tools*: Invest in a digital food scale to weigh your portions accurately, especially with calorie-dense foods like nuts, seeds, and oils. Measuring spoons and cups are also useful for quick, on-the-go prep.
- *Rely on a Nutrition App*: Apps like MyFitnessPal or Cronometer make it easy to log meals and track your macros. Input your foods to see your ratio of fats, carbs, and proteins for the day.
- *Plan Meals in Advance*: Avoid decision fatigue by pre-portioning snacks and meals ahead of time. For instance, weigh out 5-6 almonds into a snack bag for

easy grabbing or pre-make soups for lunch. A little prep ensures you stay on target without constant recalculations.
- ***Start Simple and Build Variety***: Begin with straightforward recipes, like a vegetable-based soup or steamed zucchini with olive oil. Once you're comfortable, experiment with more creative dishes using FMD-friendly ingredients.
- ***Be Mindful of Hidden Calories***: Ingredients like nuts, avocado, or olive oil are fantastic for the FMD but calorie-dense. Stick to small portions and measure carefully to avoid unintentionally exceeding your calorie target.

Examples of FMD-Friendly Foods by Macronutrient

When building your meals, focus on a balance of these nutrient-dense, low-calorie ingredients:

1. **Healthy Fats (Primary Energy Source):**
   - Olive oil (1 tsp = 40 calories)
   - Avocado (¼ avocado = 80 calories)
   - Almonds, macadamia nuts, or walnuts (6-8 nuts = approx. 100 calories)
   - Chia seeds or flaxseeds (1 tbsp = 50 calories)
2. **Low-Glycemic Carbs:**
   - Zucchini, spinach, kale, and broccoli (low-calorie and fiber-rich)
   - Cauliflower (great as a rice substitute)

- Spaghetti squash or butternut squash (small portions on Day 1)
3. **<u>Very Low Protein:</u>**
    - Tofu or small amounts of lentils (no more than ¼ cup)
    - Vegetables like mushrooms and asparagus (lower protein alternatives)

This mix supports FMD principles without overpowering your calorie limit.

The FMD isn't about obsessing over every bite. Perfection isn't the goal—consistency is. If you accidentally deviate slightly, don't give up! Focus on getting back to the plan for your next meal. Your body responds to the overall structure of the five-day cycle, and staying consistent will deliver the benefits you're aiming for.

Also, listen to your body as you adjust to the lower calorie intake. You might feel hungry on Days 2 or 3, but hydration and fat-rich snacks like a handful of nuts or herbal teas can help. Visualize how good you'll feel on Day 5, knowing that you've supported your body in profound ways.

By understanding the importance of your macro targets and using practical strategies, you'll find it easier to focus, prepare, and succeed. Stick to your plan, trust the science behind the FMD, and watch how the right combination of calories and macronutrients can transform both how you feel and how your body functions. Balance is the key to unlocking a healthier, more energized you!

Step 3: Choose the Right Foods and Supplements

Selecting the right foods is one of the most important steps when following the Fast Mimicking Diet (FMD). The goal is to choose foods that nourish your body while sticking to the diet's calorie and macronutrient guidelines. At the same time, you want to make sure your meals are enjoyable and satisfying so you can stick to the plan without feeling deprived. This step will guide you through the process, providing tips, examples, and practical advice.

Focus on Nutrient Density

When your calories are limited, every bite should count. Nutrient-dense foods are those that deliver lots of vitamins, minerals, and other important nutrients without adding too many calories. These foods help fuel your body, keep you feeling good, and make sure you're getting the most out of your meals.

What to Prioritize:

- ***Vegetables Packed with Nutrients***: Choose low-calorie, high-fiber vegetables like kale, spinach, zucchini, broccoli, mushrooms, cucumber, and celery.

These veggies not only fill you up but also provide essential vitamins and antioxidants.
- *Healthy Fats*: Incorporate small portions of olive oil, avocados, almonds, walnuts, chia seeds, or sunflower seeds. These healthy fats give you energy and keep you feeling full for longer periods. A drizzle of olive oil on a salad or a handful of walnuts as a snack can make a big difference.

Example Choices for Nutrient-Dense Foods:

- A colorful salad with mixed leafy greens, a few slices of cucumber, and a sprinkle of sunflower seeds, dressed with olive oil and lemon juice.
- Steamed broccoli or zucchini seasoned with garlic, olive oil, and a pinch of salt for a side dish packed with fiber and flavor.

Plan for Soups and Small Meals

Soups and stews are excellent meal options for the FMD because they are low in calories, easy to portion, and highly satisfying. Soups also allow you to combine several vegetables and healthy fats into one comforting dish.

Why Soups Work:

Soup keeps you hydrated because of its liquid content, which can also help curb hunger.

Pureed soups, made by blending cooked vegetables, give you a creamy, filling texture without needing high-calorie cream or butter.

How to Build an FMD-Friendly Soup:

- Start with a low-sodium vegetable broth as your base.
- Add veggies like zucchini, celery, spinach, or mushrooms for nutrients and bulk.
- Include a healthy fat source, such as a tablespoon of olive oil or avocado, to meet your macro ratios.
- Season with fresh herbs and spices such as parsley, basil, turmeric, salt, and pepper for flavor without extra calories.

Example Soups:

- A zucchini and leek soup with a drizzle of olive oil on top for a healthy lunch.
- Mushroom bisque made with pureed mushrooms, a touch of almond milk, and seasoning for a cozy dinner.

Outside of soup, light meals such as vegetable salads or stuffed bell peppers with a small amount of quinoa or lentils can offer variety while keeping you satisfied.

Consider Supplements

Supplements aren't absolutely necessary for everyone, but they can support your body during the FMD, especially if you have specific needs or are worried about nutrient gaps.

Always check with a healthcare provider before adding supplements to ensure they are right for you.

Supplement Ideas for the FMD:

- *Multivitamin*: A good multivitamin can help fill in any gaps during the five days of reduced calorie intake. For instance, if you're eating a lower amount of vegetables, a multivitamin ensures you still get enough vitamins like C, A, and B-complex.
- *Omega-3 Fatty Acids*: These healthy fats are known for their anti-inflammatory properties and overall support for brain and heart health. Consider a fish oil or algae-based omega-3 supplement if you're on a plant-based diet.
- *Electrolytes or Mineral Drops*: These can help maintain hydration and counteract fatigue, especially if you notice low energy levels. Look for low-calorie or calorie-free options.

Practical Tips to Keep You on Track

Here are additional tips to make choosing the right foods and supplements even easier during the FMD:

- *Batch Prepare Foods*: Spend an hour or two preparing soups, washing and chopping vegetables, and portioning out nuts in advance. This way, the work is done when hunger strikes.

- ***Keep Your Kitchen Tidy and Organized***: Use small containers for portioning out oils, nuts, seeds, or snacks to ensure you're eating the correct amounts.
- ***Stay Hydrated***: Drinking water consistently throughout the day can prevent dehydration and hunger pangs. Herbal teas like chamomile, ginger, or mint are great options.
- ***Don't Fear Repetition***: Repeating similar meals is fine during the FMD. Stick to easy, go-to meals that work instead of overcomplicating things with variety.

With the combination of nutrient-dense foods, satisfying small meals, and optional supplements to support your health, you can follow the FMD confidently and effectively. Planning ahead and paying attention to your portions will help you avoid pitfalls and make the process much more manageable!

Step 4: Plan Your 5-Day Cycle

Planning your five-day cycle well can make all the difference between a successful Fast Mimicking Diet (FMD) experience and one filled with uncertainty or frustration. With a little structure, meal timing, and preparation, you'll feel more in control and ready to reap the maximum benefits of the diet. Here's how to organize your days for success.

Start with a Detailed Daily Outline

Each day of the FMD is carefully designed to keep your body in a fasting-mimicking state. Structuring your days helps you stay consistent while avoiding unnecessary distractions. Here's a guideline for timing your meals and snacks:

Day 1: On this slightly higher-calorie day (approximately 1,100 calories), plan for three small meals and a snack.

Example schedule:

- *Breakfast (8 AM)*: Warm herbal tea with some nuts or seeds.
- *Mid-morning snack (11 AM)*: Broth or a nutrient-dense, low-carb soup.
- *Lunch (2 PM)*: A low-carb vegetable salad with olive oil and avocado slices.
- *Dinner (6 PM)*: Roasted zucchini with a small serving of butternut squash.

Days 2-5: These are your low-calorie days (750-800 calories). Aim for two meals per day with one snack.

Example schedule:

- *Morning drink (8 AM)*: Hot water with lemon or herbal tea.
- *Snack (11 AM)*: A small handful of nuts (5-6 almonds) or a light vegetable soup.
- *Lunch (2 PM)*: Steamed cauliflower and kale sautéed in olive oil.
- *Dinner (6 PM)*: Light broth-based soup with added zucchini or mushrooms.

Key Tips for Structuring Your Days

- *Space Out Meals Evenly*: Plan to eat every 4-6 hours to stabilize hunger and energy levels. Sticking to set meal times helps your mind and body adjust to the temporary caloric restriction.
- *Start the Day Light*: Mornings are typically when you feel less hungry, so opt for tea or warm water to ease into the day. Save your larger meals for lunch and dinner.
- *Plan Meals That Fit Into Your Lifestyle*: If mornings are hectic, prep breakfast or snacks the night before. Conversely, if you tend to have dinner with family, work around that by reserving more calories for your evening meal.
- *Hydration is Non-Negotiable*: Drink at least 8-10 glasses of water daily, plus herbal teas, to stay hydrated. This also curbs hunger and supports digestion.
- *Simplify, Don't Overcomplicate*: Stick to easy-to-prepare meals that fit within FMD guidelines. A simple soup or a handful of veggies with olive oil can satisfy you without requiring elaborate recipes.

Helpful Strategies to Stay on Track

- *Pre-Measure Portions*: Use meal prep containers to divide your day's portions in advance. This eliminates the guesswork during busy moments.

- *Create a Visual Meal Plan*: Write out (or digitally map) your five-day menu to guide you through each meal and snack. You can even pin it to your fridge as a reminder.
- *Listen to Your Body*: Hunger may come in waves, especially on low-calorie days. Combat this by sipping on warm tea, low-sodium broth, or simply distracting yourself with a light activity such as walking or stretching.
- *Avoid Triggers*: If you know certain social events or office snacks will tempt you, prepare by bringing your own FMD-friendly snacks or politely stepping away.

By building a consistent, easy-to-follow five-day plan, you'll reduce stress, stay aligned with your goals, and empower yourself to complete the FMD feeling proud and re-energized.

Step 5: Refeeding and Transitioning Back

The way you transition off the Fast Mimicking Diet is just as important as how you follow it. Proper refeeding allows your body to adjust to higher calorie and protein levels, avoids undoing your hard-earned progress, and sets the stage for long-term success. Think of this step as a continuation of your reset rather than the "end."

Start Slow on Day 6 (Refeeding Day)

Your first day post-FMD should consist of light, easily digestible meals that provide balanced nutrients. Follow these principles:

1. *Light Breakfast*: Include soft, easy-on-the-stomach foods like a smoothie or yogurt. For example:
   - Green Smoothie (spinach, unsweetened almond milk, half a banana, and a tsp of chia seeds).
   - Plain Greek yogurt with fresh berries.
2. *Nutrient-Dense Lunch*: Reintroduce small portions of protein and complex carbs along with vegetables. For instance:
   - Grilled salmon (2-3 oz) with steamed asparagus and a drizzle of olive oil.
   - Lentil soup paired with a small side of leafy greens.
3. *Gentle Dinner*: End the day with another light, nutrient-packed meal, such as:
   - Quinoa bowl with roasted vegetables and a tsp of tahini dressing.
   - Baked cod with mashed cauliflower.

Reintroduce Foods Gradually

- *Complex Carbohydrates*: Start with whole-food options like quinoa, sweet potatoes, or brown rice in small quantities (¼-½ cup per meal).

- *Lean Proteins*: Introduce proteins like salmon, chicken breast, or eggs gradually. Stick to small serving sizes (2-3 oz) on the first day post-fast.
- *Fats*: Continue incorporating healthy fats like olive oil, avocado, and nuts, as they support hormonal balance and help you feel satiated.

Avoid Common Pitfalls

- *Don't Overeat*: Your digestive system has been in a reset state. Overloading it with large or heavy meals immediately post-fast could cause bloating, discomfort, or fatigue. Listen to your hunger cues and stop eating when you're satisfied, not stuffed.
- *Skip Refined Sugars and Processed Carbs*: Reintroducing sugary or processed foods too quickly can spike blood sugar, leaving you feeling lethargic or undoing metabolic progress. Instead, stick to whole, nutrient-dense carbs.
- *Ease Back into Exercise*: Avoid jumping straight into intense workouts the day you finish the FMD. Give your body at least 1-2 days to adjust before resuming strength training or cardio. Light walking and stretching are excellent reentry options.

Extend the Benefits After Refeeding

Post-FMD, capitalize on the momentum you've built by implementing some of its core principles into your daily routine:

- *Eat More Plant-Based Foods*: Make vegetables, healthy fats, and moderate proteins a staple of your meals to support cellular health and long-lasting energy.
- *Stick to Balanced Macros*: Even outside of FMD cycles, aim for a balance of healthy fats, complex carbs, and quality proteins to keep your metabolism and hormones in check.
- *Repeat the FMD Periodically*: Depending on your goals and healthcare recommendations, consider repeating the FMD every 3-4 months to maintain its benefits. Regular cycles can help keep cellular rejuvenation and fat-burning pathways active.

Take time to reflect on how the FMD made you feel. Did it improve your energy? Help you feel more in tune with your eating habits? Use these insights to make informed decisions about your long-term wellness plan. Celebrate your commitment to your health and be proud of the investment you've made in yourself.

Transitioning smoothly out of the FMD reinforces the progress you've worked hard to achieve. By staying mindful, avoiding common pitfalls, and keeping health-promoting habits, you'll walk away not only feeling invigorated but also confident in your ability to make lasting changes. The end of the FMD isn't just a finish line; it's a gateway to a more balanced, vibrant version of you!

Supporting Hormonal Balance Through Lifestyle

Your lifestyle choices play a critical role in supporting hormonal balance and helping you get the most out of the Fast Mimicking Diet (FMD). By prioritizing sleep, stress management, light movement, and tracking progress, you can give your body the tools it needs to thrive during and after the diet cycle. Below, we'll explore actionable tips tailored to women over 40.

Sleep, Stress, and Recovery Tips

Sleep is essential for hormonal regulation, especially as your body goes through the changes of perimenopause and menopause. Poor sleep can disrupt cortisol (stress hormone) levels, insulin sensitivity, and even appetite-regulating hormones like leptin and ghrelin. During the FMD, sleep becomes even more critical because your body uses this rest period for recovery, cell repair, and regeneration.

Tips for Improving Sleep

1. ***Establish a Consistent Sleep Routine***: Go to bed and wake up at the same time every day, even on weekends. This consistency helps regulate your body's internal clock and optimizes hormonal cycles.
2. ***Create a Calming Sleep Environment***
    - Dim the lights in your bedroom an hour before bed.
    - Keep your bedroom temperature cool, around 65–68°F (18–20°C).
    - Use blackout curtains or an eye mask to eliminate light exposure.
    - Silence your phone or other devices to avoid interruptions.
3. ***Reduce Screen Time Before Bed***: Blue light from screens interferes with melatonin production, the hormone responsible for sleep. Aim to turn off electronics at least an hour before bedtime. Instead, engage in calming activities like reading or meditating.
4. ***Adopt a Relaxing Bedtime Routine***
    - Try a warm bath with Epsom salts to relax muscles and promote a sense of calm.
    - Sip on a non-caffeinated herbal tea, such as chamomile or lavender, to wind down.
    - Use calming essential oils like lavender or eucalyptus in a diffuser to ease stress.

5. ***Limit Caffeine and Alcohol***: Avoid caffeine after 2 PM and alcohol in the evening, as both can disrupt deep sleep and hormonal balance.

Stress Management Techniques

Stress triggers the release of cortisol, which can interfere with other hormones like estrogen and insulin. Chronic stress may also hinder the benefits of the FMD by increasing inflammation in the body. Incorporate these strategies to manage stress effectively:

- ***Mindfulness Practices***: Spend 10-15 minutes a day doing mindful breathing or meditation. Apps like Headspace or Calm offer guided sessions tailored to different stress levels.
- ***Gentle Yoga***: Yoga combines movement with mindfulness, making it a fantastic option for reducing stress while improving circulation and flexibility.
- ***Journaling***: Write down things you're grateful for or reflect on your emotions. Gratitude journaling has been shown to lower stress levels.
- ***Focus on Breathing Exercises***: Spend a few minutes a day practicing deep diaphragmatic breathing. Try the 4-7-8 method (inhale for 4 seconds, hold for 7, exhale for 8).

Prioritize Recovery

Recovery goes beyond rest; it's about nourishing your body and mind. On the FMD, some people may feel tired or drained. Listen to your body and prioritize recovery by:

- Napping if you feel fatigued.
- Minimizing high-stress activities or overcommitment.
- Spending time doing what you enjoy, whether it's gardening, listening to music, or reading.

Prioritizing sleep, managing stress, and focusing on recovery are essential for maintaining hormonal balance and overall well-being, especially during perimenopause, menopause, or periods like the FMD. By adopting these simple practices, you can support your body's natural processes and feel more energized and resilient.

Light Movement and Exercise Guidelines

During the FMD, your body is in a caloric deficit, so intense exercise is not recommended. Strenuous activity can increase cortisol levels and lead to unnecessary stress on your system. Instead, engaging in light movement can:

- Improve circulation and ease digestion.
- Lower stress and boost mood through endorphin release.
- Enhance joint and muscle flexibility, especially as mobility can become more challenging after 40.

Recommended Exercises During FMD

1. *Walking*: Take 20–30 minute leisurely walks around your neighborhood or in nature. Walking is a low-impact, stress-reducing way to improve circulation.
2. *Gentle Yoga*: Restorative yoga focuses on stretches and deep breathing rather than strength or intensity. Poses like Child's Pose, Cat-Cow, and Legs-Up-The-Wall are especially calming.
3. *Stretching Sessions*: Simple stretching in the morning or after meals can help release tension and improve muscle flexibility. Focus on areas like your back, shoulders, and hips.
4. *Tai Chi or Qigong*: These slow, meditative movements are great for balance, mindfulness, and relaxation.

Tips for Avoiding Overexertion

- Stay in tune with your body. If you feel fatigued or lightheaded, rest instead of pushing yourself.
- Keep movement short and gentle. Exercise sessions can be as quick as 10-15 minutes.
- Avoid high-intensity workouts like heavy weightlifting, running, or HIIT sessions during the FMD, as these may leave you feeling depleted.

Practical Tip:

Engage in movement you enjoy. Whether it's walking your dog, dancing in your kitchen, or stretching while listening to podcasts, make it something fun and stress-free.

Tracking Energy, Mood, and Progress

Tracking how you feel during and after the FMD provides valuable insights into its impact on your body. It helps you identify patterns and areas for improvement so you can adjust future cycles, ensuring a smoother and more effective experience.

What to Track

1. *Energy Levels*: Note any changes in your energy throughout the day. Do you feel more energetic in the morning? Are there specific times when fatigue sets in?
2. *Mood Changes*: Record your emotional well-being. Are you calmer, happier, or more reactive? FMD often promotes a sense of clarity and positivity, so tracking mood can confirm progress.
3. *Physical Symptoms*: Keep tabs on hunger, bloating, digestion, or any physical discomfort. These insights can help you refine food choices for future rounds of FMD.
4. *Measurements or Metrics*: If you're comfortable, document your weight, waist circumference, or other numbers to see how your body is responding.

Tools for Tracking

- *Journals*: Use a simple notebook to jot down daily observations. Split your notes into categories like "Energy," "Mood," and "Activity."
- *Apps*: Health-focused apps like MyFitnessPal or Period Tracker can monitor physical and hormonal changes.
- *Checklists*: Keep a daily checklist to note water intake, hours of sleep, and meals eaten.

Interpreting Patterns

Once you have several days or weeks of data, look for trends:

- Did your energy levels improve by Day 5 of the FMD?
- What meals made you feel fuller or more satisfied?
- How did stress levels correlate with sleep quality?

These reflections can guide you toward a more personalized approach for future FMD cycles or daily lifestyle changes.

Using Tracking Data to Stay Motivated

Celebrate small victories! Maybe your mood improved, your sleep deepened, or your clothes fit a little better. Acknowledge these gains to stay encouraged for the next round.

Supporting your hormonal balance through sleep, stress management, light exercise, and self-awareness ensures that the FMD becomes more than a temporary plan. It becomes a meaningful reset that contributes to long-term wellness for women over 40.

Sample Recipes and Meal Plan

Your meal plan is the backbone of the Fast Mimicking Diet (FMD). This chapter will provide you with sample recipes and a complete guide to stock up on essentials, follow a structured 5-day FMD plan, ease back with refeeding day recipes, and customize these to your needs. All recipes include nutritional breakdowns to align with FMD guidelines.

Key Ingredients to Stock

To succeed on the FMD, stocking your kitchen with the right foods is essential. These nutrient-dense options help keep you within caloric limits while providing the fuel your body needs.

1. **Vegetables (Low-Glycemic)**

   Choose non-starchy vegetables that help maintain stable blood sugar levels.
   - Zucchini
   - Spinach
   - Kale
   - Broccoli

- Cauliflower
- Asparagus
- Mushrooms
- Bell peppers
- Celery
- Radishes

2. **Healthy Fats**

These fats keep you full and support hormone health. Use small portions to stay within calorie limits.

- Olive oil
- Avocado
- Walnuts
- Almonds
- Macadamia nuts
- Flaxseeds
- Chia seeds
- Coconut milk (unsweetened)

3. **Complex Carbs (Use Sparingly)**

Include small amounts of these for Days 1 and 2 if allowed by your macro plan.

- Butternut squash
- Spaghetti squash
- Quinoa
- Sweet potato

4. **Broths and Herbal Teas**

   Essential for hydration and comfort.

   - Vegetable broth (low-sodium)
   - Miso broth (low-sodium)
   - Chamomile tea
   - Peppermint tea
   - Rooibos tea

5. **Other Staples**

   Enhance flavor and maintain nutrient density.

   - Sea salt and pepper
   - Turmeric
   - Cinnamon
   - Lemon juice
   - Vinegar (apple cider, balsamic, red wine)

5-Day Sample FMD Meal Plan

This 5-day meal plan is designed to provide a mix of low-calorie, nutritious meals that meet the principles of the Fast Mimicking Diet. Portions are controlled, focusing on nutrient density over volume.

Table 1: 5-Day Sample FMD Meal Plan

Day	Breakfast	Snack	Lunch	Dinner
Day 1	Warm Lemon Water + Spinach and Avocado Smoothie	5 Almonds + 1 Green Tea	Zucchini Noodles with Tomato Basil Sauce	Broccoli Soup
Day 2	Chia Pudding	5 Walnuts + Herbal Tea	Kale and Lentil Salad	Cauliflower "Rice" Stir-Fry
Day 3	Herbal Tea + Sautéed Greens with Garlic	1 Small Cucumber (with lemon)	Tofu Scramble	Creamy Roasted Cauliflower Soup
Day 4	Green Detox Smoothie	5 Almonds + Green Tea	Warm Vegetable Stew	Sweet Potato Mash Bowl
Day 5	Zucchini Fritters	1 Small Handful of Berries + Tea	Mixed Green Salad with Avocado Dressing	Cream of Mushroom Soup

Each meal and snack is intentionally light, helping your body stay in a fasting-mimicking state without overwhelming digestion. On Day 6, you can slowly reintroduce higher-calorie foods to your diet. Start with light and nutrient-dense options.

Refeeding Day Recipes

Quinoa and Veggie Bowl

Ingredients:

- ½ cup cooked quinoa
- ¼ cup steamed broccoli
- ¼ cup shredded carrots
- 2 tbsp hummus
- 1 tsp olive oil

Instructions:

1. Combine the quinoa and veggies in a bowl.
2. Add a dollop of hummus and drizzle olive oil on top.
3. Mix well and serve.

Nutrition:

- Calories: 210
- Carbs: 22g
- Protein: 6g
- Fat: 10g
- Fiber: 5g

Lentil and Sweet Potato Soup

Ingredients:

- 1 cup vegetable broth
- ½ cup cooked lentils
- ½ cup diced sweet potatoes
- Spices: thyme, paprika, garlic powder

Instructions:

1. Heat the broth in a pot and add sweet potatoes and lentils.
2. Season with spices and simmer for 10 minutes.
3. Serve warm with a squeeze of lemon.

Nutrition:

- Calories: 180
- Carbs: 30g
- Protein: 6g
- Fat: 0.5g
- Fiber: 8g

Avocado Toast with Eggs

Ingredients:

- 1 slice whole-grain bread
- ½ avocado, mashed
- 1 boiled egg, sliced
- Salt and pepper to taste

Instructions:

1. Toast the bread and spread the mashed avocado.
2. Top with sliced boiled egg and season with salt and pepper. Enjoy!

Nutrition:

- Calories: 250
- Carbs: 20g
- Protein: 10g
- Fat: 14g
- Fiber: 6g

Chickpea and Spinach Salad

Ingredients:

- ½ cup cooked chickpeas
- 1 cup fresh spinach
- 1 tbsp olive oil
- 1 tsp lemon juice
- Salt and pepper to taste

Instructions:

1. Toss cooked chickpeas and fresh spinach in a bowl.
2. Drizzle olive oil and lemon juice over the salad.
3. Sprinkle it with salt and pepper.

Nutrition:

- Calories: 200
- Carbs: 20g
- Protein: 6g
- Fat: 9g
- Fiber: 7g

Grilled Salmon with Steamed Asparagus

Ingredients:

- 1 small salmon fillet (3 oz)
- 1 cup steamed asparagus
- 1 tsp olive oil
- Lemon wedge for garnish

Instructions:

1. Grill the salmon until cooked through (about 4-5 minutes per side).
2. Steam the asparagus until tender.
3. Drizzle everything with olive oil and serve with a squeeze of lemon.

Nutrition:

- Calories: 220
- Carbs: 5g
- Protein: 23g
- Fat: 12g
- Fiber: 4g

Greek Yogurt with Berries and Nuts

Ingredients:

- ½ cup plain Greek yogurt
- ¼ cup fresh berries (strawberries, blueberries)
- 1 tbsp chopped almonds

Instructions:

1. Layer Greek yogurt in a bowl.
2. Top with fresh berries and sprinkle with chopped almonds.

Nutrition:

- Calories: 150
- Carbs: 12g
- Protein: 10g
- Fat: 7g
- Fiber: 3g

Veggie and Egg Scramble

Ingredients:

- 2 eggs
- ½ cup diced bell peppers
- ½ cup chopped spinach
- 1 tsp olive oil

Instructions:

1. Heat olive oil in a pan and sauté bell peppers and spinach.
2. Beat the eggs and pour over veggies, scrambling until cooked.

Nutrition:

- Calories: 180
- Carbs: 4g
- Protein: 14g
- Fat: 12g
- Fiber: 1g

Sweet Potato and Black Bean Bowl

Ingredients:

- ½ cup roasted sweet potatoes (cubed)
- ½ cup cooked black beans
- 1 tsp tahini
- 1 tsp olive oil

Instructions:

1. Combine roasted sweet potatoes and black beans in a bowl.
2. Drizzle with tahini and olive oil.

Nutrition:

- Calories: 210
- Carbs: 35g
- Protein: 7g
- Fat: 6g
- Fiber: 8g

Cauliflower and Kale Stir-Fry

Ingredients:

- 1 cup riced cauliflower
- ½ cup chopped kale
- 1 tsp sesame oil
- 1 tsp low-sodium soy sauce

Instructions:

1. Heat sesame oil in a pan. Add cauliflower and kale, cooking for 5-7 minutes.
2. Drizzle with soy sauce and serve.

Nutrition:

- Calories: 110
- Carbs: 8g
- Protein: 3g
- Fat: 6g
- Fiber: 3g

Roasted Vegetables with Quinoa

Ingredients:

- ½ cup cooked quinoa
- 1 cup mixed roasted veggies (zucchini, peppers, mushrooms)
- 1 tsp olive oil
- 1 tsp balsamic vinegar

Instructions:

1. Roast veggies at 375°F for 20 minutes.
2. Toss roasted veggies with quinoa, olive oil, and balsamic vinegar.

Nutrition:

- Calories: 180
- Carbs: 25g
- Protein: 5g
- Fat: 6g
- Fiber: 4g

Spinach, Mushroom and Feta Omelette

Ingredients:

- 2 eggs
- ½ cup chopped spinach
- ¼ cup sliced mushrooms
- 1 tbsp crumbled feta cheese
- 1 tsp olive oil

Instructions:

1. Heat olive oil in a non-stick pan. Sauté spinach and mushrooms until tender.
2. Beat the eggs, pour into the pan, and cook until set.
3. Sprinkle with feta cheese, fold in half, and serve.

Nutrition:

- Calories: 200
- Carbs: 3g
- Protein: 15g
- Fat: 14g
- Fiber: 1g

Baked Cod with Lemon and Garlic

Ingredients:

- 4 oz cod fillet
- 1 tsp olive oil
- 1 clove garlic, minced
- 1 tbsp lemon juice
- Salt and pepper

Instructions:

1. Preheat oven to 400°F. Place cod in a baking dish.
2. Drizzle with olive oil, sprinkle garlic, lemon juice, salt, and pepper.
3. Bake for 12-15 minutes until fish flakes easily.

Nutrition:

- Calories: 140
- Carbs: 2g
- Protein: 24g
- Fat: 4g
- Fiber: 0g

Roasted Chickpea and Veggie Wrap

Ingredients:

- ½ cup roasted chickpeas
- 1 small whole-grain tortilla
- ½ cup shredded lettuce
- ¼ cup diced tomatoes
- 1 tbsp tahini

Instructions:

1. Spread tahini on the tortilla.
2. Add roasted chickpeas, lettuce, and tomatoes.
3. Fold and serve as a wrap.

Nutrition:

- Calories: 230
- Carbs: 30g
- Protein: 8g
- Fat: 8g
- Fiber: 7g

Cucumber and Avocado Salad

Ingredients:

- 1 cup sliced cucumber
- ¼ avocado, diced
- 1 tsp olive oil
- 1 tsp vinegar
- Salt and pepper

Instructions:

1. Toss cucumber and avocado in a bowl.
2. Drizzle with olive oil and vinegar, then season with salt and pepper.

Nutrition:

- Calories: 120
- Carbs: 6g
- Protein: 1g
- Fat: 10g
- Fiber: 4g

Grilled Chicken with Mashed Cauliflower

Ingredients:

- 3 oz chicken breast, grilled
- 1 cup cauliflower florets
- 1 tbsp almond milk
- Salt and pepper

Instructions:

1. Grill chicken breast until fully cooked.
2. Steam cauliflower, then mash with almond milk, salt, and pepper.
3. Serve chicken alongside mashed cauliflower.

Nutrition:

- Calories: 180
- Carbs: 5g
- Protein: 26g
- Fat: 5g
- Fiber: 2g

Turkey and Veggie Lettuce Wraps

Ingredients:

- 3 oz cooked ground turkey
- ½ cup shredded carrots
- ¼ cup diced bell peppers
- 2 large lettuce leaves
- 1 tsp low-sodium soy sauce

Instructions:

1. Sauté turkey, carrots, and bell peppers until cooked.
2. Add soy sauce, mix, and use lettuce leaves as wraps.

Nutrition:

- Calories: 170
- Carbs: 6g
- Protein: 22g
- Fat: 6g
- Fiber: 2g

Zucchini Noodles with Pesto

Ingredients:

- 1 cup spiralized zucchini
- 1 tbsp basil pesto
- 1 tbsp grated Parmesan cheese

Instructions:

1. Lightly sauté zucchini noodles until tender-crisp.
2. Toss with pesto and sprinkle with Parmesan.

Nutrition:

- Calories: 150
- Carbs: 7g
- Protein: 4g
- Fat: 12g
- Fiber: 3g

Shrimp and Guacamole Stuffed Bell Peppers

Ingredients:

- 1 small bell pepper, halved and deseeded
- 6 cooked shrimp
- ¼ cup guacamole

Instructions:

1. Fill bell pepper halves with guacamole.
2. Top with shrimp and serve cold.

Nutrition:

- Calories: 180
- Carbs: 9g
- Protein: 16g
- Fat: 10g
- Fiber: 5g

Lentil and Kale Stew

Ingredients:

- 1 cup vegetable broth
- ½ cup cooked lentils
- 1 cup chopped kale
- 1 tbsp tomato paste

Instructions:

1. Heat broth and add lentils, kale, and tomato paste.
2. Simmer for 10-12 minutes and serve warm.

Nutrition:

- Calories: 160
- Carbs: 24g
- Protein: 9g
- Fat: 2g
- Fiber: 9g

Baked Eggplant Slices

Ingredients:

- ½ medium eggplant, sliced
- 1 tbsp olive oil
- 1 tbsp grated Parmesan cheese
- Salt and pepper

Instructions:

1. Preheat oven to 375°F. Brush eggplant slices with olive oil.
2. Sprinkle with Parmesan, salt, and pepper.
3. Bake for 15-20 minutes until golden.

Nutrition:

- Calories: 120
- Carbs: 8g
- Protein: 3g
- Fat: 9g
- Fiber: 4g

Avocado and Chickpea Toast

Ingredients:

- 1 slice whole-grain bread
- ¼ avocado, mashed
- ¼ cup cooked chickpeas
- Salt and pepper

Instructions:

1. Toast the bread and spread mashed avocado over it.
2. Top with cooked chickpeas.
3. Sprinkle with salt and pepper and enjoy.

Nutrition:

- Calories: 220
- Carbs: 25g
- Protein: 8g
- Fat: 9g
- Fiber: 7g

Stuffed Portobello Mushrooms

Ingredients:

- 2 large Portobello mushroom caps
- ¼ cup diced tomatoes
- 2 tbsp shredded mozzarella cheese
- 1 tsp olive oil

Instructions:

1. Preheat oven to 375°F. Brush mushrooms with olive oil.
2. Fill with diced tomatoes, top with mozzarella, and bake for 15 minutes.

Nutrition:

- Calories: 120
- Carbs: 8g
- Protein: 6g
- Fat: 8g
- Fiber: 2g

Lentil, Cucumber, and Dill Salad

Ingredients:

- ½ cup cooked lentils
- 1 small cucumber, diced
- 1 tsp chopped dill
- 1 tsp olive oil
- 1 tsp lemon juice

Instructions:

1. Combine lentils, cucumber, and dill in a bowl.
2. Drizzle with olive oil and lemon juice. Toss to combine.

Nutrition:

- Calories: 150
- Carbs: 22g
- Protein: 8g
- Fat: 4g
- Fiber: 9g

Grilled Zucchini with Goat Cheese

Ingredients:

- 1 medium zucchini, sliced
- 1 tbsp crumbled goat cheese
- 1 tsp olive oil

Instructions:

1. Grill zucchini slices for 3-4 minutes per side.
2. Sprinkle with goat cheese and serve warm.

Nutrition:

- Calories: 100
- Carbs: 4g
- Protein: 3g
- Fat: 7g
- Fiber: 2g

Roasted Carrot Soup

Ingredients:

- 1 cup roasted carrots
- 1 cup vegetable broth
- 1 tsp grated ginger
- 1 tsp olive oil

Instructions:

1. Blend roasted carrots with vegetable broth and ginger until smooth.
2. Heat the mixture in a pot, drizzle with olive oil, and serve.

Nutrition:

- Calories: 130
- Carbs: 19g
- Protein: 2g
- Fat: 6g
- Fiber: 5g

Turkey and Avocado Salad

Ingredients:

- 3 oz cooked turkey breast, sliced
- 1 cup mixed greens
- ¼ avocado, sliced
- 1 tsp olive oil
- 1 tsp balsamic vinegar

Instructions:

1. Arrange turkey, greens, and avocado on a plate.
2. Drizzle with olive oil and balsamic vinegar.

Nutrition:

- Calories: 180
- Carbs: 5g
- Protein: 25g
- Fat: 7g
- Fiber: 2g

Sweet Potato Breakfast Bowl

Ingredients:

- ½ cup mashed sweet potato
- 1 boiled egg, sliced
- 1 tsp tahini

Instructions:

1. Place mashed sweet potato in a bowl.
2. Add sliced boiled egg and drizzle with tahini.

Nutrition:

- Calories: 190
- Carbs: 20g
- Protein: 8g
- Fat: 8g
- Fiber: 4g

Sautéed Green Beans and Almonds

Ingredients:

- 1 cup green beans, trimmed
- 1 tbsp sliced almonds
- 1 tsp olive oil

Instructions:

1. Sauté green beans in olive oil for 5-7 minutes.
2. Sprinkle with sliced almonds and serve.

Nutrition:

- Calories: 110
- Carbs: 7g
- Protein: 3g
- Fat: 7g
- Fiber: 3g

Mediterranean Tuna Salad

Ingredients:

- 3 oz canned tuna in water, drained
- 1 cup mixed greens
- ¼ cup diced cucumbers
- 1 tsp olive oil
- 1 tsp lemon juice

Instructions:

1. Combine tuna, greens, and cucumbers in a bowl.
2. Drizzle with olive oil and lemon juice.

Nutrition:

- Calories: 150
- Carbs: 3g
- Protein: 22g
- Fat: 5g
- Fiber: 1g

Roasted Beet and Arugula Salad

Ingredients:

- 1 small roasted beet, sliced
- 1 cup arugula
- 1 tbsp crumbled goat cheese
- 1 tsp balsamic vinegar

Instructions:

1. Arrange sliced beets and arugula on a plate.
2. Top with goat cheese and drizzle with balsamic vinegar.

Nutrition:

- Calories: 120
- Carbs: 11g
- Protein: 3g
- Fat: 7g
- Fiber: 2g

Grain-Free Veggie Tacos

Ingredients:

- 4 large lettuce leaves (e.g., romaine or butter lettuce)
- ½ cup sautéed zucchini, bell peppers, and onions
- 2 tbsp mashed avocado
- 1 tsp lime juice
- Dash of paprika

Instructions:

1. Wash and dry the lettuce leaves; they will act as your taco shells.
2. Sauté zucchini, bell peppers, and onions until tender.
3. Spread a small amount of mashed avocado on each lettuce leaf.
4. Add the sautéed veggies and sprinkle with lime juice and paprika.
5. Fold the lettuce leaves and enjoy as grain-free tacos.

Nutrition:

- Calories: 180
- Carbs: 12g
- Protein: 3g
- Fat: 14g
- Fiber: 5g

Quinoa and Herb Salad

Ingredients:

- ½ cup cooked quinoa
- 1 tbsp chopped parsley
- 1 tbsp chopped mint
- 1 tbsp olive oil
- 1 tsp lemon zest
- 1 tsp lemon juice

Instructions:

1. Combine cooked quinoa, parsley, and mint in a mixing bowl.
2. Drizzle with olive oil, lemon juice, and lemon zest. Toss well.
3. Serve chilled or at room temperature for a refreshing salad.

Nutrition:

- Calories: 200
- Carbs: 20g
- Protein: 4g
- Fat: 10g
- Fiber: 3g

Vegetable Lentil Stir-Fry

Ingredients:

- ½ cup cooked lentils
- ½ cup diced carrots
- ½ cup diced bell peppers
- 1 tbsp low-sodium soy sauce
- 1 tsp sesame oil

Instructions:

1. Heat sesame oil in a skillet over medium heat.
2. Add carrots and bell peppers, stir-frying for 5 minutes.
3. Mix in the cooked lentils and soy sauce, cooking for another 2-3 minutes.
4. Serve warm as a nutrient-packed stir-fry.

Nutrition:

- Calories: 190
- Carbs: 26g
- Protein: 9g
- Fat: 5g
- Fiber: 8g

Baked Sweet Potato Wedges

Ingredients:

- 1 medium sweet potato, cut into wedges
- 1 tsp olive oil
- ¼ tsp paprika
- ¼ tsp garlic powder
- Salt to taste

Instructions:

1. Preheat the oven to 400°F.
2. Toss the sweet potato wedges in olive oil, paprika, garlic powder, and salt.
3. Arrange the wedges on a baking sheet and bake for 25-30 minutes, flipping halfway through.
4. Serve warm as a comforting side dish or snack.

Nutrition:

- Calories: 150
- Carbs: 30g
- Protein: 2g
- Fat: 4g
- Fiber: 4g

Eggplant Caponata

Ingredients:

- 1 medium eggplant, diced
- ¼ cup diced tomatoes
- 1 tbsp olives, chopped
- 1 tsp capers
- 1 tbsp olive oil
- ½ tsp oregano

Instructions:

1. Heat olive oil in a skillet. Add diced eggplant and cook until tender, about 8 minutes.
2. Stir in tomatoes, olives, capers, and oregano, cooking for another 5 minutes.
3. Serve warm or cold as a versatile side dish.

Nutrition:

- Calories: 130
- Carbs: 10g
- Protein: 2g
- Fat: 9g
- Fiber: 5g

Chickpea and Herb Couscous

Ingredients:

- ½ cup whole-grain couscous, cooked
- ¼ cup cooked chickpeas
- 1 tbsp chopped parsley
- 1 tsp tahini
- 1 tsp olive oil

Instructions:

1. Combine cooked couscous and chickpeas in a bowl.
2. Stir in parsley, tahini, and olive oil until well mixed.
3. Serve as a quick and filling refeeding meal.

Nutrition:

- Calories: 210
- Carbs: 28g
- Protein: 6g
- Fat: 7g
- Fiber: 5g

Grilled Shrimp Salad

Ingredients:

- 6 medium shrimp, peeled and deveined
- 1 cup arugula
- ¼ cup diced mango
- 1 tsp olive oil
- 1 tsp lime juice

Instructions:

1. Grill the shrimp for 2-3 minutes on each side until pink and cooked through.
2. Toss together arugula, diced mango, olive oil, and lime juice.
3. Top with grilled shrimp and serve as a flavorful salad.

Nutrition:

- Calories: 170
- Carbs: 9g
- Protein: 15g
- Fat: 7g
- Fiber: 2g

Cucumber and Tomato Salad

Ingredients:

- ½ cup diced cucumber
- ½ cup diced tomatoes
- 1 tsp olive oil
- 1 tsp balsamic vinegar

Instructions:

1. Combine diced cucumber and tomatoes in a bowl.
2. Drizzle with olive oil and balsamic vinegar; toss to coat.
3. Enjoy as a simple, refreshing salad.

Nutrition:

- Calories: 80
- Carbs: 6g
- Protein: 1g
- Fat: 5g
- Fiber: 2g

Vegetable Soup

Ingredients:

- 1 cup vegetable broth
- ½ cup diced celery
- ½ cup diced carrots
- ½ cup chopped kale

Instructions:

1. Heat vegetable broth in a pot.
2. Add celery and carrots, simmering for 10 minutes.
3. Stir in kale and cook until wilted. Serve hot.

Nutrition:

- Calories: 90
- Carbs: 12g
- Protein: 3g
- Fat: 2g
- Fiber: 4g

Healthy Berry Parfait

Ingredients:

- ½ cup plain Greek yogurt
- ¼ cup mixed berries (blueberries, raspberries, strawberries)
- 1 tbsp granola

Instructions:

1. Layer Greek yogurt in a serving glass.
2. Add berries and top with granola.
3. Serve immediately as a nutrient-dense dessert or snack.

Nutrition:

- Calories: 150
- Carbs: 15g
- Protein: 9g
- Fat: 5g
- Fiber: 3g

Tips for Customizing to Your Needs

Every woman's body is different, so tailoring the FMD to your preferences and requirements can enhance your experience.

1. **Dietary Restrictions or Allergies**
    - For vegetarians or vegans, ensure protein sources like legumes or tofu remain limited. Focus on plant-based fats and veggies.
    - For nut allergies, replace nuts with seeds such as sunflower or pumpkin seeds.
2. **Alternatives to Suit Preferences**
    - If you dislike herbal teas, try hot water with lemon or low-sodium vegetable broth as a sipping option.
    - Not a fan of certain vegetables like kale? Substitute with spinach or bok choy, ensuring nutrient density.
3. **Health-Specific Goals**
    - For weight loss, stick closely to the calorie guidelines and avoid "cheating" with high-fat or high-carb extras.
    - If blood sugar management is a focus, prioritize leafy greens and avoid starchy vegetables like carrots or sweet potatoes during the FMD.

4. **Time-Saving Tips**
    - Prep soups and snacks ahead of time to grab-and-go during busy days.
    - Double recipes to ensure leftovers for the next meal or day.

The FMD is flexible enough to accommodate individual needs while still delivering profound health benefits. Personalizing the plan will make it easier to stick with and more enjoyable to follow.

Final Tips and Encouragement

Completing your first round of the Fast Mimicking Diet is a significant achievement. It's proof of your dedication to improving your health and well-being. But the end of this cycle doesn't mean the end of your wellness journey. This chapter will give you final tips for staying motivated, listening to your body, and building a lifestyle that supports long-term balance and vitality.

Staying Motivated After the First Round

The first round is often the hardest, but it's also the most eye-opening. Now that you've completed it, staying motivated becomes easier when you focus on your progress and future goals.

1. **Celebrate Small Wins:**

    Reflect on the benefits you've experienced, whether that's more energy, better digestion, or simply the accomplishment of finishing. Write these down to remind yourself of why you started.

2. **Set New Goals:**

   Motivation thrives on having something to strive for. Whether you want to repeat the FMD quarterly, fit into a certain outfit, or increase your energy levels, having clear goals keeps you focused.

3. **Think About the "Why":**

   Revisit your reasons for starting the FMD in the first place. Was it to feel more vibrant? To improve your hormone health? Keeping your "why" front and center can reignite your drive every time you feel tempted to give up.

4. **Find a Community:**

   Surround yourself with women who share similar goals. Online forums, social media groups, or local wellness meetups can provide much-needed support and encouragement. Sharing experiences and tips can keep you inspired.

5. **Reward Yourself Smartly:**

   Treat yourself to something that aligns with your health goals, like a relaxing massage, a fitness class, or new kitchen gadgets to make meal prep easier. Positive rewards reinforce your commitment without derailing your progress.

Motivation isn't about feeling driven every moment. It's about consistently coming back to what matters, even on difficult days.

Listening to Your Body

One of the greatest tools the FMD gives you is a deeper connection to your body's signals. Learning to tune in can transform how you approach your health moving forward.

1. **Pay Attention to Hunger Cues:**

    The FMD helps reset your relationship with food, teaching you the difference between emotional cravings and physical hunger. Moving forward, pause before eating to check if you're truly hungry or just eating out of habit or boredom.

2. **Notice How Food Affects You:**

    Post-FMD, take note of how different meals make you feel. Do certain foods leave you energized, while others make you feel sluggish or bloated? Use this information to refine your regular diet to include more of what nourishes you and less of what doesn't.

3. **Tune into Your Energy Rhythms:**

    Log how your energy fluctuates throughout the day. If you feel tired after a meal or after a poor night's sleep, adjust accordingly. For example, lighter meals might work better at night, or a mindfulness practice could help you wind down before bed.

4. **Acknowledge Emotional Responses:**

    Hormonal shifts can affect your mood, stress levels, and appetite. Journaling can help identify patterns between your lifestyle choices and emotions. For example, are you more irritable when you skip self-care? Recognizing this equips you to act in a way that serves you better.

Listening to your body doesn't mean overanalyzing every sensation. Instead, it's about being mindful and using observations to make decisions that support your physical and emotional needs.

Building a Long-Term Wellness Approach

The Fast Mimicking Diet isn't just a reset; it's a foundation for long-term health. Now that you've seen what's possible, here's how to sustain and build upon these benefits over time.

1. **Adopt the FMD Principles on Non-Fasting Days:**

    Incorporate the lessons you've learned from the FMD, such as eating more plant-based meals, healthy fats, and controlling portion sizes. For example:

    - Include low-carb veggies in most of your meals.

- Replace processed snacks with nuts, seeds, or fresh produce.
- Reduce refined sugars and focus on whole, nutrient-dense foods.

2. **Schedule Periodic FMD Cycles:**

Repeating the FMD every few months (as recommended by your healthcare provider) can help maintain the benefits you've built, such as improved metabolism and hormonal balance. Treat it as an ongoing tool in your wellness toolbox.

3. **Prioritize Holistic Health:**

Diet is just one pillar of health. Ensure your lifestyle also supports wellness in other areas:

- Stress: Incorporate daily stress-reducing practices, such as yoga, meditation, or a gratitude journal.
- Sleep: Stick to routines that prioritize restorative rest.
- Exercise: Aim for a mix of strength, cardio, and flexibility exercises.

4. **Stay Flexible:**

Your body, schedule, and goals will evolve over time. What worked for you today might not work as well in six months. Be open to adjusting your lifestyle so it continues to meet your needs.

5. **Focus on Consistency, Not Perfection:**

   Building a wellness approach isn't about perfect adherence every day. It's about consistently making choices that move you closer to your goals. Celebrate progress, not perfection, to sustain a positive and sustainable mindset.

By turning the FMD into a stepping stone for broader wellness habits, you'll create a lifestyle that supports energy, hormonal balance, and vitality for years to come.

Conclusion

Taking control of your health after 40 doesn't have to feel like an uphill battle. The Fast Mimicking Diet (FMD) offers a powerful, scientifically-backed way for you to reset your body, support hormonal balance, and promote longevity without giving up food entirely. By completing just five days of low-calorie, nutrient-rich meals, you can tap into remarkable benefits like improved energy, mental clarity, and sustainable weight management. More importantly, the FMD equips you with a deeper understanding of your body's needs, making it a sustainable tool for both short-term resets and long-term health.

One of the most important takeaways from the FMD is its ability to help you address the hormonal shifts that inevitably come with aging. If you've been feeling fatigued, struggling with stubborn weight gain, or navigating the brain fog of perimenopause or menopause, the FMD works to give your body the reset it craves. By promoting processes like autophagy, ketosis, and reduced inflammation, it supports cellular rejuvenation and hormonal harmony, leaving you feeling more in control of your health.

But the benefits don't stop there. The FMD isn't just about fixing what's out of balance; it's about enhancing what already works. During those five days, you're not just eating fewer calories; you're fueling your body with clean, plant-based foods packed with nutrients. You're teaching your system to burn fat more effectively and reducing markers of aging like insulin resistance and IGF-1 levels. By the end of the diet, most women experience not only weight loss but also improved digestion, sharper mental clarity, and a noticeable boost in energy.

What makes the FMD particularly powerful is its sustainability. It's not another restrictive, all-or-nothing diet that leaves you burnt out and frustrated. Instead, it's a tool you can integrate periodically to maintain your progress and keep building toward better health. By scheduling regular FMD cycles, you give your body the periodic break it needs to repair, rejuvenate, and recalibrate. Plus, the principles of the diet, such as reducing sugar and prioritizing healthy fats, can be seamlessly applied to your everyday life for long-term results.

If you're hesitating to jump in, remember this: the FMD is a commitment of just five days, with results that can transform how you feel for weeks or even months after. It's an excellent starting point for anyone looking to overcome common challenges in their 40s and beyond, from hormonal imbalances to reduced energy. Better yet, it's backed by science and supported by countless women who have used it to reclaim their health and confidence.

Now's the time to act. Whether it's your first FMD cycle or your fifth, each round is an opportunity to invest in yourself, reset your system, and align with the vibrant, balanced health you deserve. Take those first steps today by preparing your pantry, setting your intentions, and embracing a plan designed to support you—not just for five days, but for life. You're stronger than you think, and with the FMD, achieving your health goals is well within reach.

FAQs

Can I Do This Monthly?

Yes, many women incorporate the FMD monthly as a part of their wellness routine. The typical recommendation is to complete one five-day cycle every 3-6 months, but some individuals, especially those seeking metabolic resets or weight loss, may benefit from doing it monthly. Always consult your healthcare provider to ensure it aligns with your personal health needs.

Is It Safe During Perimenopause?

Absolutely. The FMD is designed to support hormonal balance, making it particularly beneficial during perimenopause when estrogen, progesterone, and insulin sensitivity fluctuate. By promoting fat-burning, reducing inflammation, and improving insulin sensitivity, the FMD helps manage many symptoms like weight gain, fatigue, and brain fog. However, it's best to check with your doctor before starting, especially if you have other medical conditions.

What If I Feel Fatigued During the Fast?

Feeling tired during the FMD is normal, particularly on Days 1-2 as your body shifts into a fasting-like state and begins burning fat for energy. To manage fatigue:

- Stay hydrated and sip on herbal teas or broth.
- Rest when needed and avoid intense exercise.
- Supplement with electrolytes like magnesium or potassium to reduce fatigue.
- If fatigue feels extreme, consult your doctor and consider adjusting your approach.

Who Should Avoid the FMD?

The FMD is not suitable for everyone. Women who are pregnant, breastfeeding, underweight, or have a history of eating disorders should avoid it. Additionally, those managing serious medical conditions such as diabetes, heart disease, or undergoing cancer treatment must consult their physician before attempting the diet.

What Are the Benefits for Women Over 40?

The FMD offers multiple advantages, including supporting hormonal balance, promoting fat loss, reducing inflammation, improving mental clarity, and enhancing energy levels. It also rejuvenates cells through autophagy and can help reduce the risk of chronic diseases like heart issues or Type 2 diabetes, which are more common as we age.

Do I Need to Buy Special Products for the FMD?

Not necessarily. While there are pre-packaged FMD kits available, many women prefer to follow the guidelines with whole, store-bought foods. Stock up on nutrient-dense, low-calorie options like leafy greens, nuts, seeds, vegetable broths, and healthy fats to create meals tailored to the diet. Prepping your pantry in advance is key to success.

How Do I Transition Back to Normal Eating After the FMD?

Refeeding after the FMD is crucial. On Day 6, stick to light meals like soups, steamed vegetables, and small amounts of protein to allow your digestive system to adjust. Gradually reintroduce complex carbohydrates and heavier protein meals over the following days. Avoid jumping into heavy or processed foods to maintain the progress you've achieved.

References and Helpful Links

Crider, C. (2024, June 20). What is a fasting mimicking diet? Healthline. https://www.healthline.com/nutrition/fasting-mimicking-diet

Newcomb, B. (2024, November 6). Fasting-Like diet lowers risk factors for disease, reduces biological age in humans. USC Leonard Davis School of Gerontology. https://gero.usc.edu/2024/02/20/fasting-mimicking-diet-biological-age/

Lucchetti, L. (2024, January 17). The Fasting-Mimicking Diet: A Guide. Healthgrades. https://resources.healthgrades.com/right-care/food-nutrition-and-diet/fasting-mimicking-diet

Furthermore from Equinox. (n.d.). https://fm.equinox.com/articles/2020/02/fasting-mimicking-diet#:~:text=While%20you%20can%20take%20part,create%20stem%20cells%2C%20Foroutan%20says.

Howley, E. K., & Burdeos, J. (2024, April 25). What is a Fasting-Mimicking Diet? US News & World Report. https://health.usnews.com/wellness/food/articles/what-is-the-fasting-mimicking-diet

Burkhart, A. (2025, March 18). Fasting mimicking diet (Prolon): What is it? Does it work? Amy Burkhart, MD, RD. https://theceliacmd.com/fasting-mimicking-diet-what-is-it-does-it-work/

R, S. (2023, April 19). Fast mimicking diet recipes. Shakthi Health & Wellness. https://www.raowellness.com/fast-mimicking-diet-recipes/

www.ingramcontent.com/pod-product-compliance
Lightning Source LLC
LaVergne TN
LVHW012027060526
838201LV00061B/4496